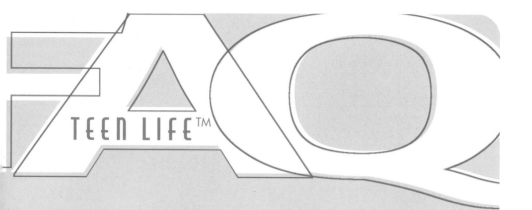

TEEN LIFE™

FREQUENTLY ASKED QUESTIONS ABOUT

Cosmetic
Surgery

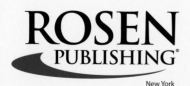

Nellie Vlad and
Frances O'Connor

ROSEN
PUBLISHING®

New York

Published in 2012 by The Rosen Publishing Group, Inc.
29 East 21st Street, New York, NY 10010

First Edition

Library of Congress Cataloging-in-Publication Data

Vlad, Nellie.
Frequently asked questions about cosmetic surgery/
Nellie Vlad, Frances O'Connor.—1st ed.
    p. cm.—(FAQ, teen life)
Includes bibliographical references and index.
ISBN 978-1-4488-5559-9 (lib. bdg.)
1. Surgery, Plastic—Popular works. I. O'Connor, Frances. II. Title.
RD118.V53 2012
617.9'52—dc22

                                        2011012011

Manufactured in China

CPSIA Compliance Information: Batch #W12YA. For further information, contact Rosen Publishing, New York, New York, at 1-800-237-9932.

What Distinguishes Cosmetic Surgery from Plastic Surgery and Reconstructive Surgery?

Most plastic surgery developments occurred in the early twentieth century, during World War I (1914–1918). For the first time, surgeons saw many terrible facial and head injuries, which were caused by weapons such as poison gas, machine guns, and grenades. These wounds challenged surgeons to develop new skills and procedures. By the 1950s and 1960s, doctors had learned to do breast jobs and tummy tucks. Liposuction (the removal of excess fat from under the skin by suction) was developed in the 1970s.

The American Society of Plastic Surgeons (ASPS), a leading authority on information about cosmetic and reconstructive plastic surgery, is an organization of board-certified plastic surgeons. It is also the only organization that has compiled cosmetic and plastic surgery statistics and information over more than twenty years. According

WHAT DISTINGUISHES COSMETIC SURGERY FROM
PLASTIC SURGERY AND RECONSTRUCTIVE SURGERY?

5

to the ASPS, there are differences between cosmetic surgery, plastic surgery, and reconstructive surgery:

• **Cosmetic surgery** is surgery that is performed to reshape normal structures of the body. For instance, there may not be anything medically wrong with your nose, but you want to have cosmetic surgery so that your nose looks more attractive to you.

• **Plastic surgery** is surgery dealing with the repair of injured, deformed, or destroyed parts of the body. Often this surgery involves transferring skin and bone from other parts of the body or from another person. For example, someone who was in a car accident may have sustained extensive injury to his or her face. A plastic surgeon might take pieces of bone from another part of the person's body to reconstruct a damaged cheekbone and jaw.

• **Reconstructive surgery** is a type of plastic surgery. It is performed on abnormal structures caused by congenital defects (defects that you were born with), developmental defects, trauma (as a result of an accident), infection, tumors, or disease.

Teens are the most controversial new kind of cosmetic surgery patient. Although the majority of cosmetic surgery patients aren't teenagers, according to the ASPS, more teens are getting cosmetic surgery than ever before. In 2009, nearly 210,000 cosmetic surgery procedures (including minimally invasive

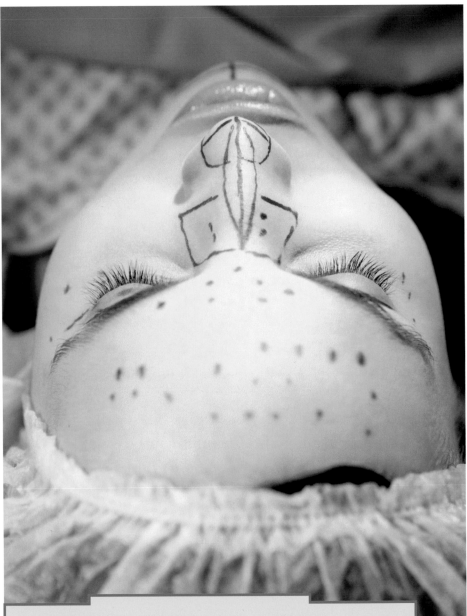

A young woman is being prepared for cosmetic surgery. According to the ASPS, 91 percent of the 12.5 million cosmetic procedures performed in 2009 were done on women.

WHAT DISTINGUISHES COSMETIC SURGERY FROM
PLASTIC SURGERY AND RECONSTRUCTIVE SURGERY?

7

procedures) were performed on young people between the ages of thirteen and nineteen. In this age group, thirty-five thousand patients had nose reshaping (rhinoplasty). That's nearly 50 percent of all cosmetic surgery procedures performed on people in this age group (almost seventy-five thousand). According to the ASPS, a total of 13.1 million Americans had cosmetic surgical procedures in 2010 (this total includes minimally invasive surgery). This figure is up 5 percent from 2009 (12.5 million).

With the growth of such a trend comes an increase in the concerns adults have about teen cosmetic surgery. Researcher Kearney Cooke said, "What's most disturbing to me is that this is a time when their bodies aren't fully formed, yet teens feel so much pressure to be instantly perfect."

The top five cosmetic surgical procedures performed on teens ages thirteen to nineteen in 2009, with the most popular listed first, were nose reshaping, breast reduction in men, breast augmentation, ear surgery, and liposuction. Most teens who want to have cosmetic surgery often have it to improve some physical characteristic that they believe makes them imperfect or awkward. They think that if they don't have the physical characteristic corrected, the imperfection will follow them into adulthood—they want to fit in, not stand out from their peers. Many adults, on the other hand, have cosmetic surgery done to stand out from other people.

Not every person who wants to have cosmetic surgery is right for the procedure. People need to understand the benefits and the risks. They need to have realistic expectations about the operation and what it can do for them. Most doctors will expect certain growth benchmarks to have been achieved by a teen before even considering him or her as a possible candidate for cosmetic surgery.

Most health insurance plans will not cover cosmetic surgeries; however, many plans will provide coverage if a cosmetic procedure relieves physical symptoms or improves the way a person's body works. Nevertheless, health insurance coverage varies widely among health plans. Cosmetic surgery is something not to rush into. You'll need to think carefully about what is involved in surgical procedures; what to expect before, during, and after the operation; and what are possible complications and recovery and healing issues. Find out all the facts about cosmetic surgery before making a decision.

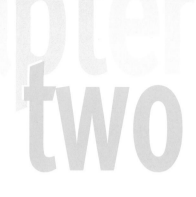

What Are Some Common Cosmetic Surgery Procedures?

Nationwide, the most popular cosmetic procedure is breast augmentation. Other popular procedures include nose reshaping, eyelid surgery, liposuction (also called lipoplasty), tummy tucks, and face-lifts. Also high on the list are laser hair removal, chemical peels, skin resurfacing, dermabrasion and microdermabrasion skin work, pinning back ears, and penile enlargement.

Breast Augmentation

Breast augmentation surgery is one of the most popular surgeries for teens. According to the ASPS, this surgery decreased in popularity by 9 percent from 2008 to 2009. However, with a reported 8,199 breast augmentation surgeries performed on young women between the ages of eighteen and nine-

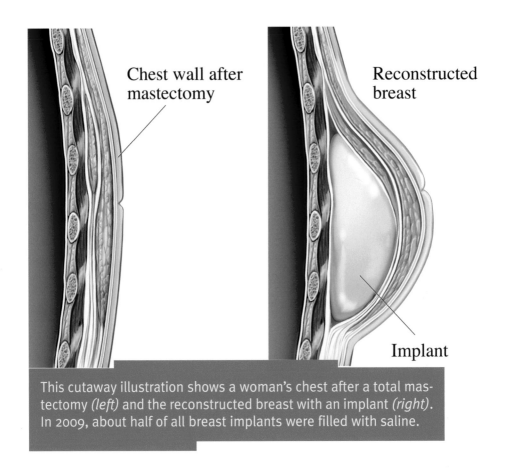

Chest wall after mastectomy

Reconstructed breast

Implant

This cutaway illustration shows a woman's chest after a total mastectomy *(left)* and the reconstructed breast with an implant *(right)*. In 2009, about half of all breast implants were filled with saline.

teen in 2009, it's still in the top five cosmetic surgeries for this age group.

At first, breast implants were used mostly for breast cancer patients who had mastectomies. Many of the early breast implants, those done in the 1960s, used an implant that was a rubber silicone envelope filled with silicone gel. Only about 10 percent were filled with saline (salt water). In 1992 the U.S. Food and Drug Administration (FDA) banned the use of silicone breast implants after studies found a possible link between leaking silicone and autoimmune diseases. It was thought that if a silicone breast implant broke, the leaking silicone would invade the surrounding tissue and harden, and the body would attack its own cells. On November 17, 2006, the FDA approved the return of silicone breast implants manufactured by Allergan Corporation and Mentor Corporation after reviewing extensive data from clinical trials of women who had the implants. About the FDA ruling, Dr. Daniel Schultz, director of the FDA's Center for Devices and Radiological Health, said, "The extensive body of scientific evidence provides reasonable assurance of the benefits and risks of these devices. This information is available in the product labeling and will enable women and their physicians to make informed decisions."

Today, most breast implants are saline-filled implants because many doctors still prefer to use them, citing less risk to their patients in the event of a rupture or leak. In January 2011, the FDA raised the possibility of a link between anaplastic large cell lymphoma (ALCL) and breast implants. ALCL is a rare type of non-Hodgkin's lymphoma, a cancer involving the cells of the immune system. According to National Cancer Institute studies, 1 in 500,000 women is diagnosed with ALCL in the United States annually. Based on reported cases of ALCL in women with breast implants, there was a possible association between the implants and ALCL, although the occurrence was low. Currently, the FDA is unable to identify a specific type of implant that is associated with a lower or higher risk of ALCL. In the cases linked to implant patients, the lymphoma, which is not breast cancer, grew in the breast, often in the capsule of scar tissue around the implant. In some cases, just removing the implant and scar tissue seemed to eliminate the disease.

Nose Reshaping

Rhinoplasty is the name cosmetic surgeons gave to nose reshaping. This is the most common aesthetic procedure requested by teens, according to the ASPS. The nearly thirty-five thousand teens who had nose reshaping in 2009 made up 14 percent of the seventy-five thousand having cosmetic surgical procedures in the thirteen- to nineteen-year-old age group. Rhinoplasty can be performed when the nose has completed 90 percent of its growth, which can occur as young as age thirteen or fourteen in girls and fifteen or sixteen in boys. There are a number of rhinoplasty procedures. Surgeons can shave off a bone to get rid of a bump, place nasal implants to lengthen the nose, cut wide nostrils, raise the tip of the nose, get rid of a hooked nose, and/or reshape the nose bridge.

How is it done? First, the doctor separates the skin of the nose from the underlying bone and cartilage. The bone and cartilage are then reshaped, and the skin is redraped over the surface. Sometimes the bone is broken, but that is not as common as it used to be.

Eyelid Surgery

Blepharoplasty, or eyelid surgery, is a common cosmetic procedure performed on many teenagers. In 2009, there were 1,892 teens, ages thirteen to nineteen, who had eyelid surgery. This procedure extends the eyelid, giving the patient a more wide-eyed appearance. Many people think that this wide-eyed look makes a person appear younger, fresher, and smarter. The procedure is performed by making cuts in the natural contour lines of the upper eyelid.

Liposuction

There were 3,179 teens between the ages of thirteen and nineteen who had liposuction operations in 2009, according to the ASPS. Liposuction is a procedure that sucks the fat out of a part of the body. How is this done? Usually, the doctor begins the surgery by draw-

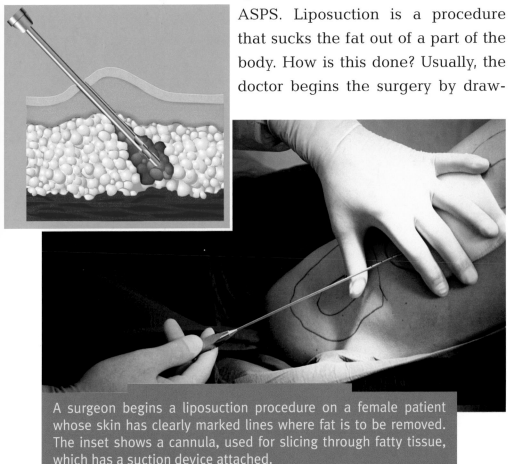

A surgeon begins a liposuction procedure on a female patient whose skin has clearly marked lines where fat is to be removed. The inset shows a cannula, used for slicing through fatty tissue, which has a suction device attached.

ing lines on the patient's skin to mark where the fat is to be removed, and then the patient is put under general anesthesia. Sometimes the doctor runs an ultrasound wand over the site of the liposuction to liquefy the fat. That makes the fat easier to remove. The doctor then inserts a tube about the size of a ball-point pen into the site and vacuums the fat into a beaker.

In tumescent liposuction, also called "wet" liposuction, the doctor floods the fat with fluids. This makes the suction easier and lets the doctor take out more fat. The fluid contains epinephrine (adrenaline), which constricts blood vessels and reduces bleeding. It also contains lidocaine, an anesthetic, which gives enough pain control that a patient may not need general anesthesia.

Tummy Tuck

Abdominoplasty, more commonly called a tummy tuck, is a surgical procedure during which excess skin and fat are removed from the abdomen. Muscles also may be tightened. A horizontal cut is made in the abdomen at the level of the pubic hair. The excess abdominal skin and fat above the incision are then dissected away from the muscles. The abdominal muscles are tightened with stitches. The two skin edges are brought back together, which creates a flatter abdomen because a segment of the skin and fat was removed. The navel remains in the same place but must be brought out through another opening in the skin. That means that the navel gets covered over with skin when the skin shifts during the operation. To make the navel visible again, the doctor has to cut a hole in the skin covering the navel and pull it from under the skin to the top layer of the skin, where it can be seen again. Liposuction of the hips often is performed with abdominoplasty. The ASPS reported that there were 116,000 tummy tuck procedures performed in the United States in 2010.

Dermabrasion and Dermaplaning

Dermabrasion is the process of scraping away the outer layers of skin. It is a procedure often done to correct acne scars or other scarring and to remove fine wrinkles. Dermaplaning is a surgical technique that is usually used to treat scarring from deep acne and uses a handheld instrument known as a dermatome. A dermatome looks something like an electric razor with an oscillating blade that moves back and forth to cut thin slices off the surface layers of skin. In dermabrasion, surgeons use a rough wire brush or burr that contains diamond particles and that is attached to the high-speed motorized handle of a surgical tool. The tool scrapes away or "sands" the skin until the level of skin is reached that will make a scar less visible. This is done to allow new skin to grow. According to the ASPS, 2,721 teens (ages thirteen to nineteen) had dermabrasion procedures in 2009.

Hair Removal by Laser

Laser hair removal is a procedure by which hair is removed from the body with a long pulse laser. A trained laser specialist or doctor focuses the light of the long pulse laser onto an area of skin and holds it there. Depending on which area of your body— whether your arm, bikini line, or upper lip—the laser applies a different strength of light and pulse duration to match the depth, size, and location of the follicle (root).

Laser hair removal works by disabling hair in its active growth cycle, and deadens the follicle to stop hair from growing back. Because different parts of the body have hair that enters growth cycles at different times, several treatments are usually necessary to make sure that the laser has caught new growth before it can continue.

The FDA doesn't allow doctors or treatment centers to advertise that they remove hair 100 percent effectively for life, so most advertisements for this procedure will read "high success rate" or up to 90 percent removal. In 2009, there were 65,308 teens, ages thirteen to nineteen, who had laser hair removal procedures, according to the ASPS.

Ear Surgery

Otoplasty, or ear pinning, is a popular surgery for children and teens. This surgery can be performed on anyone six years or older. It may require a stay in the hospital, or it may be done in a doctor's office. The risks of the procedure, however, are the same as for any surgery.

During this procedure, cuts are made behind the ears to lay open the ear cartilage. The doctor can then stitch the cartilage together or can remove excess cartilage. Lastly, the doctor stitches the skin of the ears into place. There were 7,909 teens (ages thirteen to nineteen) who had otoplasty procedures in 2009, as reported by the ASPS.

Phalloplasty

Phalloplasty, or penis enlargement, is done to accomplish two goals. The first goal is to make the penis appear longer. Penile lengthening procedures usually make the penis appear noticeably longer only in its flaccid (soft) state. The second goal is to make the penis wider.

There are some experimental techniques used to increase the width of the penis. Some of these techniques include injecting fat from other parts of the body into the penis, or carving strips of fat from a person's buttocks or thighs and then injecting them into cuts made in the shaft of the penis. Some men try to increase the width of the penis by getting collagen injections, even though collagen can cause allergic reactions.

How is penile lengthening done? The surgeon snips the suspensory ligament, which attaches the base of the penis to the pubic bone. The "inner penis" is then tugged away from the bone. Once the wound heals, the penis hangs lower.

Breast Reduction

Both women and men get breast reductions, or breast mammoplasties, as surgeons call them. Breast reductions are performed when a person's breasts are unusually large for his or her body.

TECHNIQUES

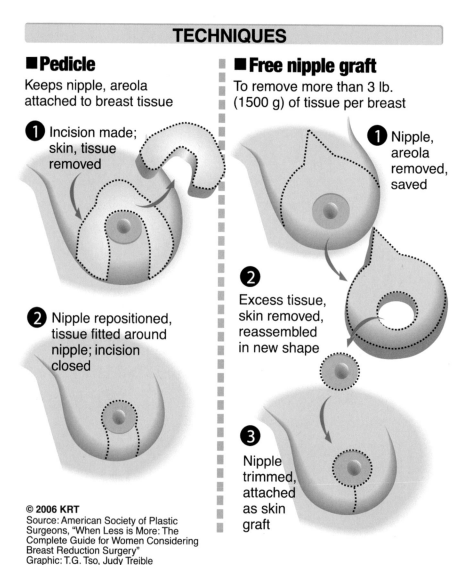

■ Pedicle

Keeps nipple, areola attached to breast tissue

1 Incision made; skin, tissue removed

2 Nipple repositioned, tissue fitted around nipple; incision closed

© 2006 KRT
Source: American Society of Plastic Surgeons, "When Less is More: The Complete Guide for Women Considering Breast Reduction Surgery"
Graphic: T.G. Tso, Judy Treible

■ Free nipple graft

To remove more than 3 lb. (1500 g) of tissue per breast

1 Nipple, areola removed, saved

2 Excess tissue, skin removed, reassembled in new shape

3 Nipple trimmed, attached as skin graft

These illustrations show two popular techniques for breast reduction surgery. Of the 78,427 breast reduction procedures done in 2009 on men and women, 4,346 were performed on teens between the ages of thirteen and nineteen, as stated by the ASPS.

The breast reduction procedure removes fat and glandular tissue—and in some cases, excess skin—from the breasts, leaving them smaller and more firm.

When men have large breasts, the condition is called gynecomastia. The word "gynecomastia" comes from a Greek word meaning "women-like breasts." According to the ASPS, it's quite a common condition, affecting an estimated 40 to 60 percent of men. Many of them choose to have a breast reduction. In 2009 alone, a reported seventeen thousand men in the United States had gynecomastia reduction surgery. There were 12,908 gynecomastia operations performed on teens, ages thirteen to nineteen, in 2009—that represents 75 percent of the total for that cosmetic surgical procedure.

Face-lift

The medical term for a face-lift is rhytidectomy. This surgical procedure removes excess fat, tightens underlying facial muscles, and redrapes the skin of the face. It does not improve the appearance of sagging eyelids or foreheads, or baggy neck skin, so many people have surgery on these areas as well as getting a face-lift. The ASPS reported that in 2009, 103,625 Americans got face-lifts. The gender distribution for that total was 94,029 women and 9,596 men.

A face-lift is done by making cuts above the hairline at the temples, extending the cut in front of the ear or inside the cartilage at the front of the ear, and then continuing behind the earlobe to the lower scalp. Then the surgeon separates the skin from the fat and muscle below. Fat can be trimmed or sucked from around the neck and chin. The surgeon then tightens the underlying muscle and pulls the skin back, removing the extra skin. This gives facial skin a tighter appearance. After the surgery, a small tube may be temporarily placed under the skin behind the ear to drain any blood that might collect there. The surgeon also may wrap the head with bandages to try to minimize the bruising and swelling.

Cosmetic Minimally Invasive Procedures in High Demand

Sometimes people feel that while their face doesn't need drastic reshaping, they are not pleased with how their skin appears. In these cases, they may look for procedures that are minimally invasive, meaning they barely invade, or go below, the skin's surface. This can help to correct common problems such as dry skin, sagging skin, or acne scars. As plastic surgeons perform more surgeries, they find ways to treat problems without having to go below the skin and cause trauma to a large area of tissue. Owing to their work and that of researchers over the past ten years, many new procedures have been developed.

Botox

Botox is a trade name for *botulinum toxin A*, which is a bacterium that blocks the signals that would normally tell your muscles to contract. In performing this procedure, the doctor injects a small amount of the *botulinum toxin A* into a muscle

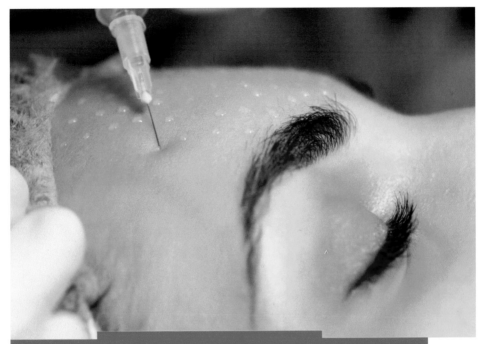

A doctor injects a patient's forehead with Botox. Botox, which is made from the bacterium *botulinum toxin A*, temporarily causes muscle relaxation and is commonly used to treat facial wrinkles.

group to paralyze this area and make wrinkles and frown lines "disappear" for a period of three to eight months. Botox is injected into the face and neck to paralyze muscles and reduce the signs of aging, such as sagging and wrinkles. It is not yet recommended by doctors or approved by the FDA for injection in other areas of the body for cosmetic purposes. In 2010, Botox procedures were the most popular minimally invasive cosmetic procedures performed in the United States, numbering 5.4 million, according to the ASPS.

Chemical Peel

A chemical peel is a procedure usually used to improve the appearance of the skin of the face, neck, or hands. The doctor applies a combination of chemical solutions—usually an alpha hydroxy acid, such as glycolic acid, salicylic acid, or lactic acid; trichloroacetic acid (TCA); or carbolic acid (phenol)—to the skin to make it blister and eventually peel off within a few days to two weeks. The period of time it takes the acid to produce peeling depends on how concentrated the solution is and how much is applied. This chemically burned skin gives way to new, regenerated skin that is usually smoother and less wrinkled than the old skin. The procedure causes a warm, burning sensation and requires pain medication to treat the wounds as they heal. The ASPS reported that more than 1.1 million Americans had chemical peels in 2010.

Microdermabrasion

The microdermabrasion procedure is sometimes called a "mini-peel." The procedure is meant to remove the signs of dry skin, acne scars, and enlarged pores and to improve blood circulation to the surface of the skin. It is a surgical technique that doctors use to abrade the skin with a high-pressure flow of crystals. The procedure was first developed in Italy in 1985. Microdermabrasion is now popular in the United States because it has the advantage of being a low risk procedure with a quick recovery compared with other skin resurfacing procedures. It involves using aluminum oxide crystals to finely resurface the layers of the skin as it exfoliates. The crystals move over the surface of the skin, sort of polishing it. In the process, it removes the surface scarring that is caused by acne, for example. You may have to return for a few treatments to see a significant reduction in acne scars or sun damage, as microdermabrasion only takes care of the skin's topmost layer. According to the ASPS, 9,563 teens between the ages of thirteen and nineteen had microdermabrasion proce-dures done in 2009.

Plumping

Plumping is the common name for soft tissue filler injections, such as collagen, into certain parts of the body. The lips often receive this treatment to make them appear fuller. Collagen is a liquid made from the connective tissue of cows or pigs. Injectable collagen is used for filling in "contour deformities" in the skin, such as acne scars or wrinkles. It is injected beneath the skin of the part of the body that is being "plumped." Though the procedure is commonly done, the FDA has not approved the use of collagen for enlarging facial features, such as lips. The ASPS reported that in 2010, there were 1.8 million Americans who had soft tissue filler injection procedures.

Myths and Facts

 A doctor's office is a safer environment than a hospital's surgical room because the doctor pays close attention to you in his or her office.

Fact: ➡ Doctors' offices often don't have up-to-date equipment or the equipment needed if there was a complication during the procedure.

 Only women and girls have cosmetic surgery procedures.

Fact: ➡ According to the ASPS, a reported 1.1 million male patients underwent cosmetic surgery procedures in 2009.

 Botox isn't really a serious cosmetic procedure.

Fact: ➡ Though it's not surgery, Botox injections are still a procedure, which means that it is a lot more complicated than, say, getting your teeth cleaned. The risks associated with Botox, which is a strain of botulism poison, are: 1) prolonged paralysis of tissues in the affected area; 2) if an injection is given improperly, Botox can stray to other areas of the face or body; 3) serious bacterial infection if too much of the botulinum toxin A is given.

three

Why Do People Get Cosmetic Surgery?

Why do people want to have cosmetic surgery? A quick look at some of the most popular procedures shows that the main reason why people get cosmetic surgery is because they are dissatisfied with their appearances. People get fat removed (liposuction) from every area of the face and body that you can name: they get fat sucked from under their eyes to make the bags under their eyes go away. They get the fat sucked from under their cheekbones to make their cheekbones more defined. They get fat sucked from their abdomens to get rid of a spare tire or love handles. Many young people get breast augmentation, or breast implants. Any surgery, however, comes with a set of risk factors.

A Trendy Option for Teens with Hang-ups?

It has long been known that the teenage years have been tied to a heightened concern with physical appearance and body image. "Teenagers who are thinking about having plastic surgery to change the way they look are often addressing issues of self-esteem," said psychotherapist Dorothy Ratusny in "Bodies Under Construction," an article posted on Fazeteen .com. In the same article, Dr. Darrick Antell, a New York City plastic surgeon, said that he has seen a greater number of teen patients, partly because there has been an increase in the visi-

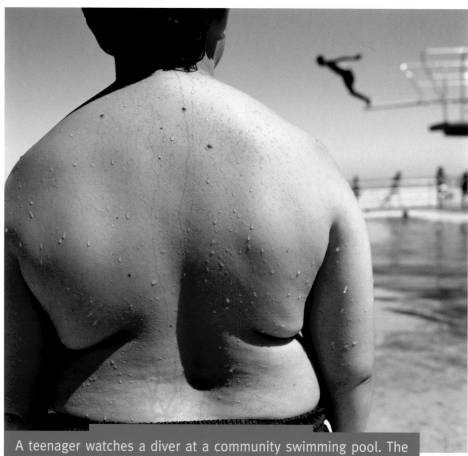

A teenager watches a diver at a community swimming pool. The teen years are challenging for many because they struggle with body image issues and self-esteem. Some teens think that cosmetic surgery can help make them look "perfect."

bility of cosmetic surgery. Antell said, "Today's teenagers are growing up with parents who have had cosmetic surgery, so they see and hear about it more. The media has also done a good job of making people aware of the procedures available. Another reason is acceptability."

In 2010, in a *Science Daily* article about research linking reality television and cosmetic surgery, Charlotte Markey, a psychology professor at Rutgers University in Camden, New Jersey, said that teens are affected by reality TV programs that "tout happiness as just a nip/tuck away." Markey's research found that young women were more likely to want cosmetic surgery than men after viewing cosmetic surgery shows. For young bodies and minds still in development, she says these drastic decisions may have implications long after their high school years. Markey said, "What troubles me is that there's no conclusive data that cosmetic surgery even makes people happier. What has been documented is that it makes repeat customers."

People want to improve their appearance because they may believe their flaws are worse than they actually are. In its most severe form, this is called body dysmorphic disorder, but people's perception of their appearance may have nothing to do with the way others see them. Instead, it may have more to do with the advertising with which individuals are surrounded every day. Consider the advertisements, for example, on television, in magazines, and on billboards that use beautiful people to sell products. These advertisements increase the chance that someone who looks fine, who is perfectly fit, could feel dissatisfied with his or her body.

Remember, too, that the cosmetic industry is a big business. Many companies have lots of money invested in fueling unrealistic expectations of how people should look. Therefore, the message is everywhere. Turn on the television and there are numerous advertisements for gyms and weight-loss programs. Turn on the radio and the same commercials are there. It is hard to escape the media blitz telling you that you should look different from how you do.

The Need to Be Beautiful and Thin

One big reason why people have cosmetic surgery is that they want to be attractive, whatever that means to them. They want

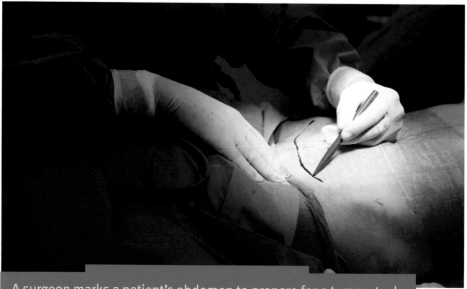

A surgeon marks a patient's abdomen to prepare for a tummy tuck. The ASPS reported that nearly 115,000 people had abdominoplasty procedures in the United States in 2009.

luscious lips like their favorite movie star, so they get collagen injected into their lips. They want a flatter stomach, so they get a tummy tuck. Another reason is that people want to be thin. This is an especially dangerous part of body image because the desire to be thin has caused near-epidemic proportions of eating disorders, as well as terrible cosmetic surgery disasters.

Some people get cosmetic surgery because they want to express themselves, and they do so by altering their appearances. Body modification has gotten much attention in recent years. It is important to remember, in this looks-conscious society, that real health may have little to do with what people see as the appearance of health or beauty. If you have ever considered cosmetic surgery, ask yourself what the main reason is. Chances are that you may feel the need to reach some standard of beauty that is totally unrealistic and that has little to do with health.

Cosmetic Surgery and the Role of Parents

If it is your parents who are suggesting that you have cosmetic surgery, ask them what their reasons are for wanting you to have it. Dr. Edward Domanskis, a surgeon who has a personal Web site where he conducts online consultations with patients, said that he receives a lot of e-mail from teenagers inquiring about cosmetic surgery. He said, "In our society, there is no such thing as being too thin. A preoccupation with the body and a constant focus on small flaws can become an obsession with teens." Nor is it just the teenagers themselves who may have

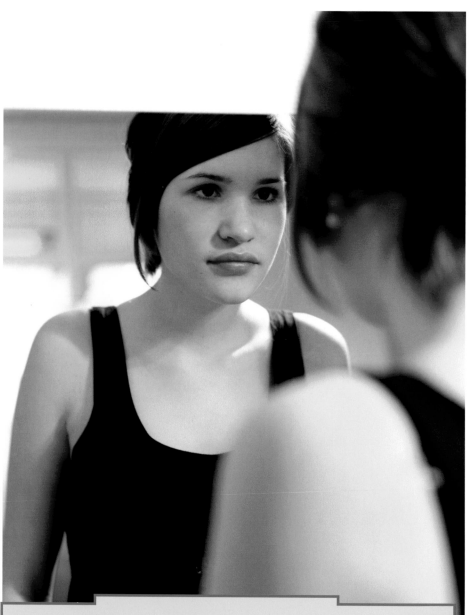

One reason why a young woman might want to have breast augmentation surgery is because of extreme breast asymmetry. Another might be because a parent is pushing her to have the surgery.

the idea to get plastic surgery. Domanskis recalled the case of a nineteen-year-old woman who came to a cosmetic surgeon for breast augmentation. After consultation, it was clear that it was the woman's mother who wanted her daughter to get the surgery so that the daughter's breasts would match her sister's. The doctor performed the surgery, but the mother was still unsatisfied, and so the girl went through another procedure. Many doctors must question, when faced with a prospective client who is a teenager, who really wants the surgery—the child or the parent.

four

What Are Some Major Issues to Keep in Mind About Cosmetic Surgery?

First, you should be aware that not all of the people performing cosmetic surgery procedures are experienced in doing them. Second, you should know that the risks become real far more often than anyone realizes. This is because many of the procedures are done in doctors' offices, not in hospitals, and the statistics are not reported. Third, you should not believe that the newer, "safer" cosmetic surgery techniques mean that cosmetic surgery is safe. The risks of surgery are always present, no matter how evolved the new techniques are.

Cost Is a Consideration

The risks go beyond the immediate physical danger. Cosmetic surgery is expensive, and because it is elective surgery, many health insurance companies do not cover the costs. That means consumers must pay out of their own pockets. Cosmetic surgery can run into the thousands of dollars, and many people finance the surgeries no matter what the cost. According to figures published in the 2009 ASPS physician fees document, the national average of surgeons/physicians' fees for the most popular five procedures were: $2,769 for liposuction; $4,936 for a tummy tuck; $4,216 for nose reshaping; $3,331 for breast augmentation; and $2,809 for eyelid surgery.

Surgeons' Advertisements

What is the role of advertising in cosmetic surgery? Advertisements not only entice people to get a procedure done,

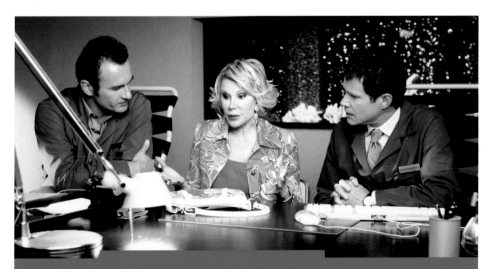

Comedian Joan Rivers appeared on the TV drama *Nip/Tuck* as a character wishing to have all her cosmetic surgeries reversed for her grandson so that he would learn that people don't have to be perfect.

but they also convey the general tone that more plastic surgery is better. This is dangerous because the more procedures that are done, the longer you are on the operating table, and the greater the risk. "There's a considerable amount of deception and outright fraud by doctors whose greed far exceeds their scruples and surgical skills," said Dr. Mark Gorney, former president of the ASPS. "Patients pay with their looks, sometimes even their lives, because a slick ad lures them into the wrong hands." Cosmetic surgery is even being auctioned off on the Internet. In fact, the state of California is so worried about sleazy advertising campaigns that it passed a law in 2000 banning inflated credentials, false scientific claims, deceptive before-and-after pictures, misleading testimonials, and statements that downplay the risks and pain of procedures. As part of this law, doctors may not claim they are "board certified" unless they specify which board certified them.

Certification

The American Board of Plastic Surgery is a member board of the American Board of Medical Specialties. There are specific and detailed training procedures that plastic surgeons must go through before they can qualify for board certification. That means that, before becoming certified, plastic surgeons must have graduated from an accredited medical school; completed at least six years of surgical training, with a minimum of three years in plastic surgery; and passed written and oral tests to prove that they have understood the training and can perform

WHAT ARE SOME MAJOR ISSUES TO KEEP IN
MIND ABOUT COSMETIC SURGERY?

35

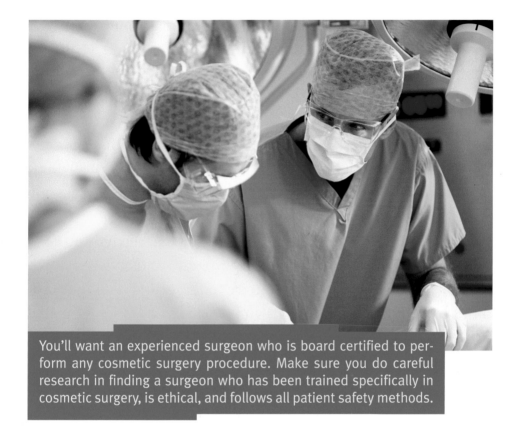

You'll want an experienced surgeon who is board certified to perform any cosmetic surgery procedure. Make sure you do careful
research in finding a surgeon who has been trained specifically in
cosmetic surgery, is ethical, and follows all patient safety methods.

the procedures of plastic surgery. The American Board of Plastic
Surgery is one of twenty-four accredited specialty boards recog-
nized by the American Board of Medical Specialties.

Once a certificate from the American Board of Plastic
Surgery is obtained, it must be renewed every ten years. This is
to make sure that plastic surgery practitioners keep up-to-date
with the newest and safest medical technology. For this reason,
it's very important to ask doctors from which board they've
received certification. Not all doctors receive certificates from an
accredited board.

Patients can have a hard time sorting out who is and is not board certified. "This is confusing for the public," said Dr. Russel Palmer, past president of the Plastic Surgery Society's Broward County, Florida, chapter. "Many people want to call themselves 'board-certified' plastic surgeons and so they create their own board. It's troubling."

There is no one organization that exists to monitor the problems with cosmetic surgery, which can potentially add to the confusion. Instead, the American Board of Plastic Surgery, the American Board of Facial Plastic and Reconstructive Surgery, the American Society of Plastic Surgeons, and the American Society for Aesthetic Plastic Surgery together regulate the standards of cosmetic surgery.

The Decision-making Process and Medical Malpractice

Except in the case of an emergency, a doctor must obtain a patient's agreement for any course of treatment. The ASPS calls the physician-patient relationship one of shared decision-making, or informed consent. Doctors must tell the patient anything that would affect the patient's decision. Informed consent varies from state to state, but generally the doctors explain the nature of the treatment, its risks, side effects, results, and other courses of action that are reasonable. Some states let older minors give consent to certain procedures.

Medical malpractice is negligent behavior by a doctor or other health care provider. A doctor's behavior is considered

WHAT ARE SOME MAJOR ISSUES TO KEEP IN
MIND ABOUT COSMETIC SURGERY?

37

negligent when he or she fails to follow accepted professional standards of care, and that care, or lack of it, causes harm to the patient.

People to Ask About Cosmetic Surgery

If you are thinking about cosmetic surgery, it's best to ask a few people for advice. Ask your parents or other adults you trust who can help you figure out if the change you're looking for is an emotional one or a much-needed physical solution. Also, ask a board-certified plastic surgeon who will give you an honest answer about

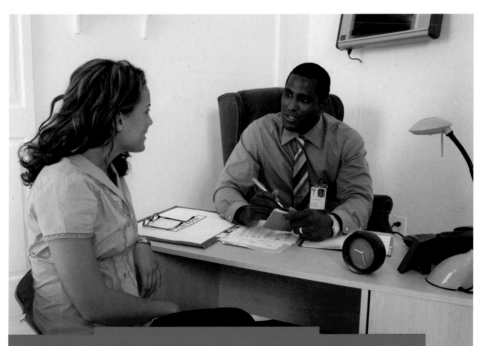

If you have questions about a cosmetic surgery procedure, ask a surgeon who is certified by the American Board of Plastic Surgery. A knowledgeable surgeon can help you evaluate your reasons for seeking surgery.

the surgery and its benefits as well as risks to your health. The ASPS (http://www.plasticsurgery.org) provides a brochure, "Make the Right Choice," to offer people information about procedure expectations and to answer general questions about cosmetic surgery. Make sure you don't ask an unqualified doctor whose answer might be motivated by the amount of money he or she will charge you.

Also keep in mind that procedures like nose reshaping can be performed only when the nose has completed 90 percent of its growth. (This can occur by age thirteen or fourteen in girls and a year later in boys.) In the case of breast augmentation or reduction, according to the ASPS, it's best to delay surgery until breast growth ceases to get the best results. With all procedures, however, it's important to consult a board-certified plastic surgeon and ask for his or her opinion regarding your age and if your body is ready for a procedure.

Ten Great Questions to Ask a Doctor

 1 Are there cosmetic surgery standards?

 2 What does it mean if a doctor says he or she is board certified?

3 How do I know what I'm agreeing to when I consent to cosmetic surgery?

4 What is medical malpractice?

5 Should I talk to people who have already had cosmetic surgery to see if they're pleased with the results?

 6 How will a cosmetic surgery procedure affect me if I haven't finished growing?

7 How long will it take to heal after the procedure?

8 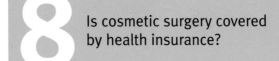 Is cosmetic surgery covered by health insurance?

9 What if one of my parents suggests I have cosmetic surgery?

10 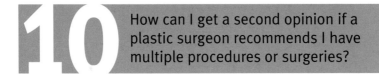 How can I get a second opinion if a plastic surgeon recommends I have multiple procedures or surgeries?

What Are the Risks and Dangers of Cosmetic Surgery?

Cosmetic surgery procedures claim to enhance attractiveness in an almost magical fashion. Doctors, and even spas, that perform many cosmetic procedures advertise cosmetic surgery as though it is no more difficult, painful, time consuming, or expensive than getting a facial. However, cosmetic surgery is a surgical procedure like any other, and as with any surgical procedure, there are risk factors.

It is important to review the risks of any surgery, as well as the risk factors specific to each cosmetic procedure. These risk factors are a result of the surgical techniques used, the process of the surgery, and the areas of the body on which the work is being done.

In the *Gale Encyclopedia of Medicine*, the risks of cosmetic surgery are described as the following:

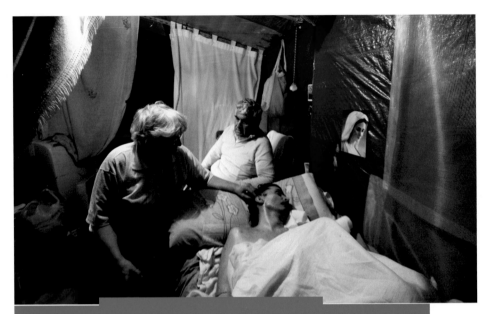

Parents take care of their son in a homemade shelter. The son went to a hospital for a simple nose operation, but when the anesthesiologist was called away, no one saw the oxygen tube slip from his mouth. He has been in a coma for twenty-one years.

- Wound infection
- Internal bleeding
- Pneumonia
- Reactions to the anesthesia
- Formation of undesirable scar tissue
- Persistent pain, redness, or swelling in the area of surgery
- Anemia (lowering of the red blood cell count, which makes a person very weak)
- Fat embolisms (when fat cells travel through the body and lodge somewhere) from liposuction
- Rejection of skin grafts or tissue transplants

• Loss of normal feeling or function in the area of operation
• Complications resulting from unforeseen technological problems

In addition, some of the other complications of cosmetic surgery—and any surgery—include the following:

• Crusting along the incision lines. After surgery, some fluid drains from a wound, which is normal. However, if it doesn't go away at the rate of a normal scab (depending on size, from one to two weeks), it can signal an infection.
• Numbness. Small sensory nerves under the skin are occasionally cut when the incision is made or interrupted by undermining of the skin during surgery. Sometimes the sensitivity never returns.
• Abnormal scars. Sometimes scars—which usually take a year or longer to fade completely—fail to heal. Injection of steroids into the scars, placement of silicone sheeting onto the scars, or further surgery to correct the scars may be necessary.
• Injury to deeper structures, such as blood vessels, nerves, and muscles.
• Medical complications such as pulmonary embolism (blockage by a blood clot of an artery in the lung), severe allergic reactions to medications, cardiac arrhythmia (irregular heart beat), heart attack, and hyperthermia (uncontrollable fever) are some of the serious and life-threatening risks of cosmetic surgery

and any surgery you might have. No one knows how often cosmetic surgery proves fatal because risk data are not compiled in a central clearinghouse.

Besides all of the general risks associated with any surgery, you should be informed—and should ask—about specific risks associated with the particular surgery you are considering. For example, phalloplasty carries with it a risk of decreased erections and permanent penile deformity.

A Riskier Choice: Outpatient Cosmetic Surgery

Many patients find that the promise of outpatient surgery is more comforting than a hospital stay. However, it is the outpatient surgery that can be riskier. Remember that hospitals are required to meet strict equipment and personnel guidelines. That may not be the case with a doctor's office. In fact, in 1999, the New York State Senate Committee conducted an investigation of cosmetic surgery performed in offices rather than in hospitals. What the committee found was shocking: compared to a hospital or an ambulatory surgical center, an office is the most dangerous place in which to undergo anesthesia. Anesthesia equipment in offices is frequently out-of-date or poorly kept. In fact, some physicians purchase old anesthesia machines for their offices, which have been discarded by hospitals because they are not up to code.

Furthermore, laws differ from state to state. In New York, for example, any person with a medical license can advertise that

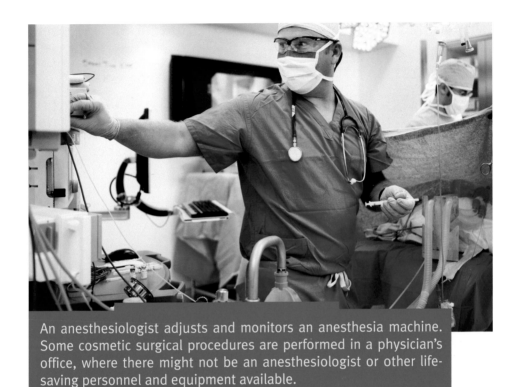

An anesthesiologist adjusts and monitors an anesthesia machine. Some cosmetic surgical procedures are performed in a physician's office, where there might not be an anesthesiologist or other life-saving personnel and equipment available.

they do liposuction or perform other cosmetic procedures. Some doctors may perform such procedures with no more preparation than a three-day weekend seminar or a thirty-minute video-taped training session. There have been numerous stories of cosmetic surgery patients who suffered serious complications or even died because the doctors' offices did not have the equipment that was needed to save their lives.

If cosmetic surgery is being performed in a doctor's office, there might not be an anesthesiologist, although anesthesia should be given only by a trained anesthesiologist. Even with an anesthesiologist, anesthesia can be tricky. Brain damage, nerve damage, eye damage, stroke, burn, myocardial infarction (irreversible injury to the heart muscle), and death can all result from incorrectly administered anesthesia.

Some Risks Linked to Common Procedures

Some of the risks associated with common procedures are listed below. You may be surprised to find that even quick, in-office procedures can result in serious complications.

Abdominoplasty

With tummy tuck surgery, you run the risk of blood clots, infection, bleeding under the skin, and poor healing resulting in noticeable scarring or skin loss. Blood clots are what happen

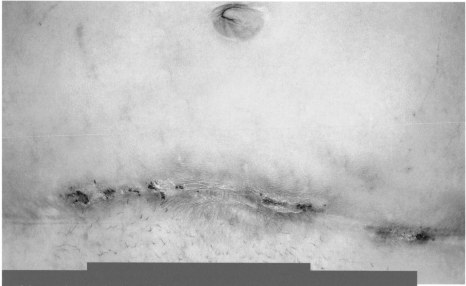

This patient's incision from a tummy tuck procedure became infected and still shows signs of an infection one year after the operation.

when blood coagulates, or thickens. Blood clots can lodge in a part of the body and block off the supply of blood or oxygen to that part, resulting in a host of problems. In addition, you can contract necrotising fasciitis, a potentially fatal infection. There also is a very slight risk of peritonitis, an inflammation that occurs if the abdominal muscle gets punctured.

Blepharoplasty

The risks of eyelid surgery include hemorrhage (heavy or uncontrollable bleeding), infection, unfavorable external scarring, blindness, ectropion (retraction of the lower lid), persistent dry eyes, irritation in the cornea, not enough skin left (meaning you must get a skin graft), asymmetry, sensitivity to light, numbness, itching, and reaction to medications.

Breast Augmentation

Any breast augmentation poses the risk of asymmetry, meaning that the breasts could be two different sizes and you will have to undergo surgery again to make them look symmetrical. Persistent pain is another potential complication. A thick scar, also called a capsule, can form around the implant as part of the body's normal reaction to a foreign substance. When the scar becomes firm, or hardens, it is called capsular contracture. This may cause pain. It may also change the texture and appearance of the breast.

Implants, which are usually filled with saline, can also rupture and leak. They can deflate, or they can become displaced. The chances of capsular contracture or rupture increase with the age of the implant. If one of these complications occurs, you will have to have outpatient surgery to loosen the capsule or remove or replace the implant.

Other risks include joint pain and swelling, skin tightness, swelling of hands and feet, rash, swollen glands or lymph nodes, unusual fatigue, general aching, viruses and flu, unusual hair loss, memory problems, headaches, muscle weakness or burning, nausea or vomiting, irritable bowel syndrome, and a greater chance of getting colds. In addition, all implants must be removed or replaced after a number of years. The amount of time an implant lasts in your body varies from person to person, but the FDA has found that by the time a woman has had implants for ten years, at least one of them has broken.

When getting a mammogram, which is used to test for breast cancer or any other illness or abnormality in the breast tissue, women have to get a special kind of mammogram to move implants away from the breast tissue. It is important to remember that implants can interfere with detecting breast cancer by "hiding" a suspicious lesion, or spot. Also, it may be hard for the doctor reading the mammogram to tell whether there is a tumor or if it is calcium deposits that formed in the scar tissue from the breast implant.

There can be either temporary or permanent change or loss of sensation in the nipple or breast tissue. Silicone has been linked to increased symptoms for connective tissue diseases such as arthritis or lupus.

Removing Upper Layers of the Skin

In dermabrasion, the patient must avoid direct sunlight for six to twelve months while the skin's pigmentation (coloring) returns.

There is the danger of permanent skin color changes, infection, scarring, flare-up of skin allergies, fever blisters, and cold sores. The smoothing effects of the surgery are said to be permanent, but they do not prevent new skin eruptions from forming. In some cases, heart irregularities could occur.

Liposuction

The liposuction procedure has some risk. "To put it in perspective," said Robert del Junco, former president of the California State Medical Board in an October 2000 article in *People* magazine, "The incidence of death from liposuction is two to three times higher than that of dying from a normal pregnancy." According to the FDA, in a paper updated in March 2010, some studies show that the risk of death due to liposuction is about 3 deaths per every 100,000 procedures, whereas other studies indicated that the risk of death is between 20 and 100 deaths per 100,000 liposuction procedures. As reported in the FDA's article, "One study suggests that the death rate is higher in liposuction surgeries in which other surgical procedures are also performed…One paper compares the deaths from liposuction to that for deaths from car accidents (16 per 100,000)."

Patients often donate their own blood prior to liposuction surgery in case a transfusion is required. You could have difficulty breathing during or even after the surgery. The cause could be anything from an allergic reaction to heart failure. In addition, sometimes pieces of fat can break off and float through the bloodstream. This is called a fat embolus, and it poses many of the same health risks that blood clots do.

You run the risk of infection, clots, fluid accumulation, skin loss, perforation of organs, pain, swelling, bleeding, numbness, rippled or baggy skin, uneven pigmentation, asymmetry, and scarring. Liposuction can cause fluid buildup in the lungs and fatal blood clots. Also, patients can lose too much fluid during the suctioning process, sending them into shock.

Some fluid that is pumped into the body during wet liposuction is suctioned back out with the fat, but most is absorbed into your blood. This can result in congestive heart failure and pulmonary edema (fluid in the lungs), both potentially fatal. Finally, one of the risks of wet liposuction is that too much epinephrine can be flooded into your system, which could lead to cardiac arrest.

Penile Enlargement

In phalloplasty, the loss of support from when the ligament is cut can lower the angle of the erection. The newly exposed shaft portion of the penis may be covered by unwanted pubic hair. The ligament can reattach to the pubic bone and retract (pull back) the penis farther inside than it was before. Other complications may include infection, scarring, cosmetic deformity, sexual dysfunction, and shrinkage. "Penile augmentation procedures are unsafe, primarily because the outcome is unpredictable and any patient can end up with a shorter penis instead of a longer penis," said Dr. Jack McAninch, former president of the American Urological Association. He also said that "deformities are significant [and] the scarring that results is significant."

The American Urological Association has declared fat injection and cutting the suspensory ligament in the penis neither safe nor effective. The American Society for Aesthetic Plastic Surgery says that penile fat injection is experimental, with "insufficient data to establish its safety and effectiveness."

Collagen Injection

The use of collagen injections (plumping) has been associated with connective tissue diseases such as lupus and scleroderma, as well as polymyositis and dermatomyositis, where the body's immune system begins to fight against itself, mistaking its own cells for foreign bodies. The FDA is still investigating how often people get connective tissue diseases after getting collagen injections.

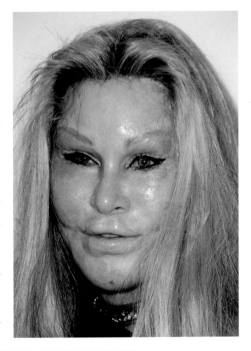

It is possible that you could be allergic to collagen and not even know it. Reactions could take the form of a rash, hives, joint and muscle pain, and headaches, and severe reactions that include shock and

Jocelyn Wildenstein, a socialite, has had many cosmetic surgeries, including rhinoplasty, chin implants, and face-lifts. Most people believe she's someone who has had excessive cosmetic surgery.

difficulty breathing. Other bad effects that have occurred after collagen injections include infections, abscesses, open sores, lumps, peeling of the skin, scarring, recurrence of herpes simplex, and partial blindness.

Reduction Mammaplasty

Breast reduction surgery, although beneficial for some people, also carries many risks. As with breast augmentation, there is a chance that the breasts will be asymmetrical. Swelling, pain, and bruising are temporary results, but can last for as long as six months. The extent of scarring depends on each person's body, but is a permanent result for every surgery patient, and it can be extensive. Hematomas (collection of blood under the skin), seromas (collection of fluid under the skin), nerve damage, and infections are possible risks of breast reduction surgery.

One unpredictable result of this kind of surgery is the possible loss of the ability to breast-feed, which you can only be sure of after a pregnancy when you try to breast-feed for the first time. For many women, this gamble is enough to dissuade them from getting the surgery. To best ensure the ability to breast-feed in the future, you should ask your surgeon to preserve milk-producing tissue and not to sever the nipple completely during surgery.

Rhinoplasty

As with any surgery, there is a risk of infection in nose reshaping. The sensation in your nose could be permanently altered, or it could be lost altogether. There could be breathing obstruction, in which case you would have to undergo another surgical procedure so that you can breathe again. There could also be nasal septal perforation (a hole in your septum). There is a risk of swelling, bruising, discomfort, infection, and scarring. The swelling may not go down for months after the surgery. Moreover, there is no guarantee that the results will be symmetrical.

Rhytidectomy

As with any cosmetic surgery, there are risks involved with getting a face-lift. These risks include reactions to anesthesia such as problems breathing, cardiac arrest, and death. Bleeding, infection, hematoma, and injury to the nerves that control facial muscles can also occur.

Before Moving Ahead

Teens and their parents need to keep in mind that surgeries are never risk-free. Before moving ahead with any kind of cosmetic surgery, they should research the procedure thoroughly, reading up on the complications and risks that are involved. Another aspect to keep in mind is nonsurgical options for changing a person's body image, for example, through exercise and a healthy diet.

Plastic surgery can be positive under the right circumstances, especially if a teen is seeking cosmetic surgery to correct a noticeable physical defect or to improve the body's function. Young adults who are part of the decision-making process can make responsible choices if they are informed and have the

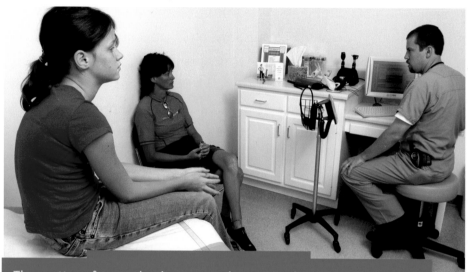

The matter of teens having cosmetic surgery is very controversial. Make sure you are well-informed and are not resorting to a procedure just to combat bullying by your peers.

physical, emotional, and mental maturity to understand what it is that they wish to achieve, set realistic expectations, understand the procedures' risks, complications, and treatment concerns, and the long-term physical effects of these cosmetic surgeries.

abrade To scrape or wear away by friction or erosion.

abscess A swollen, inflamed area of the body in which pus gathers.

accredited Furnished with credentials; licensed.

anesthesia Medicine used to produce numbness, loss of feeling, or unconsciousness.

blood clot A lump formed when blood coagulates, or sticks together.

body dysmorphic disorder A disorder in which people obsess about small flaws on their bodies.

breast augmentation A procedure, also known as augmentation mammoplasty, to enlarge the breasts, typically consisting of inserting a silicone bag under the breast or under the breast and chest muscle, and then filling the bag with saline (salt water). The silicone bag expands the breast area to give a fuller breast.

cardiac arrest When the heart stops beating.

cardiac arrhythmia An abnormal heartbeat caused by heart disease and high blood pressure.

cartilage Tough tissue in the body of which structures like the ears and the nose are partially made.

collagen The major structural protein found in animal connective tissue, yielding gelatin when boiled.

congenital Present from birth.

dermabrasion A technique for removing the upper layers of skin.

epinephrine A hormone secreted by the adrenal gland that increases heart rate and muscular strength.

exfoliate To come apart or be shed from a surface in scales or layers; to scrub skin with a gritty substance to remove the dead surface layer.

face-lift Surgery performed to remove sagging skin and wrinkles from a patient's face.

general anesthesia Anesthesia given by injection to induce a loss of consciousness.

hematoma When blood collects at a surgical site.

lidocaine A type of anesthesia.

mastectomy Surgery to remove a breast.

minimally invasive surgery Surgery that is performed with only a small incision or no incision at all, such as that performed with a laparoscope or endoscope.

oscillating Moving or swinging back and forth at a regular speed.

peritonitis Inflammation of the peritoneum, the smooth membrane that lines the cavity of the abdomen.

pulmonary thromboemboli Common complication caused when blood clots lodge in the lungs.

reconstructive surgery Correction of an abnormality caused by birth defects, disease, or traumatic injury.

suspensory ligament A ligament suspending an organ or part.

ultrasound wand A tool that uses ultrasonic waves (waves of a frequency so high that humans can't hear them), sometimes for the purposes of surgery.

American Academy of Dermatology (AAD)

P.O. Box 4014

Schaumburg, IL 60168-4014

(866) 503-SKIN (7546)

Web site: http://www.aad.org

The AAD advances the diagnosis and cosmetic treatment of
the hair, skin, and nails. Its Web site's resources include
fact sheets, a glossary of dermatological terms, and other
informational materials.

American Academy of Facial Plastic and Reconstructive
Surgery

310 South Henry Street

Alexandria, VA 22314

(800) 332-FACE (3223) or (703) 299-9291

Web site: http://www.aafprs.org

This society promotes the highest quality facial plastic surgery through education, research, and the establishment
of professional standards.

American Board of Plastic Surgery, Inc.

Seven Penn Center, Suite 400

1635 Market Street

Philadelphia, PA 19103-2204

(215) 587-9322

Web site: http://www.abplsurg.org

The American Board of Plastic Surgery promotes safe, ethical, and effective plastic surgery by maintaining high standards for the education, examination, certification, and recertification of plastic surgeons. Its Web site includes information for consumers, including answers to frequently asked questions.

American Society for Aesthetic Plastic Surgery (ASAPS)

Find-a-Plastic-Surgeon Referral Service

Web site: http://www.surgery.org

This source offers information on cosmetic surgery procedures and patient safety and a "before and after" photo gallery. You can also find statistics and news releases, and search for a surgeon in your area.

American Society of Plastic Surgeons (ASPS)

Plastic Surgery Educational Foundation

444 E. Algonquin Road

Arlington Heights, IL 60005

(847) 228-9900

Web site: http://www.plasticsurgery.org

The mission of the ASPS is to advance quality care by encouraging high standards of plastic surgery training, ethics, physician practice, and research. Its Web site includes news on the latest advances and techniques, plus information on specific procedures and a directory to help find a plastic surgeon in your region.

Canadian Dermatology Association (CDA)

1385 Bank Street, Suite 425

Ottawa, ON K1H 8N4

Canada

(613) 738-1748 or (800) 267-3376

Web site: http://www.dermatology.ca

The CDA represents Canadian dermatologists and aims to advance the science and art of medicine and surgery related to the care of the skin, hair, and nails.

Canadian Society for Aesthetic Plastic Surgery (CSAPS)

2334 Heska Road

Pickering, ON L1V 2P9

Canada

(905) 831-7750

Web site: http://csaps.ca

The CSAPS is the only professional organization in Canada dedicated to improved cosmetic surgery outcomes through education, research, and the maintenance of high surgical standards of clinical practice.

Web Sites

Due to the changing nature of Internet links, Rosen Publishing has developed an online list of Web sites related to the subject of this book. This site is updated regularly. Please use this link to access the list:

http://www.rosenlinks.com//faq/csurg

For Further Reading

Bailey, Kristen. *Cosmetic Surgery* (At Issue Series). Farmington Hills, MI: Greenhaven Press, 2005.

Espejo, Roman. *Cosmetic Surgery* (Opposing Viewpoints). Farmington Hills, NY: Greenhaven Press, 2011.

Espejo, Roman. *The Culture of Beauty* (Opposing Viewpoints). Farmington Hills, MI: Greenhaven Press, 2009.

Farndon, John. *From Laughing Gas to Face Transplants: Discovering Transplant Surgery* (Chain Reactions). Chicago, IL: Heinemann-Raintree, 2007.

Gay, Kathlyn. *Body Image and Appearance: The Ultimate Teen Guide* (It Happened to Me). Lanham, MD: The Scarecrow Press, 2009.

Kirberger, Kimberly. *No Body's Perfect: Stories by Teens About Body Image, Self-Acceptance, and the Search for Identity*. New York, NY: Scholastic, 2003.

Kotler, Robert. *The Essential Cosmetic Surgery Companion: Don't Consult a Cosmetic Surgeon Without This Book!* Beverly Hills, CA: Ernest Mitchell Publishers, 2005.

Lankford, Ronnie D., Jr. *Body Image* (Hot Topics). Farmington Hills, NY: Lucent Books, 2010.

Lusted, Marcia Amidon. *Cosmetic Surgery* (Essential Viewpoints). Edina, MN: ABDO Publishing Company, 2010.

Margolis, Leslie. *Fix*. New York, NY: Simon & Schuster Children's Publishing, 2006.

Olesen, R. Merrel, and Marie B. V. Olesen. *Cosmetic Surgery for Dummies*. Hoboken, NJ: Wiley Publishing, 2005.

Palad, Thea. *Mixed Messages: Interpreting Body Image and Social Norms* (Essential Health: Strong Beautiful Girls). Edina, MN: ABDO Publishing Company, 2009.

Perry, Arthur. *Straight Talk About Cosmetic Surgery*. New Haven, CT: Yale University Press, 2007.

Rinzler, Carol Ann. *The Encyclopedia of Cosmetic and Plastic Surgery* (Facts on File Library of Health and Living). New York, NY: Facts on File, 2009.

Walsh, Marissa. *Does This Book Make Me Look Fat? Stories About Loving—and Loathing—Your Body*. New York, NY: Clarion Books, 2008.

Willett, Edward. *Negative Body Image* (Danger Zone: Dieting and Eating Disorders). New York, NY: Rosen Publishing, 2007.

Williams, Mary E. *Self-Mutilation* (Opposing Viewpoints). Farmington Hills, MI: Greenhaven Press, 2007.

Index

A

advertising, 16, 27, 28, 33–34, 41, 44–45
Allergen Corporation, 11
alpha hydroxy acid, 22
American Board of Facial Plastic and Reconstructive Surgery, 38
American Board of Medical Specialties, 34, 35
American Board of Plastic Surgery, 34, 35, 36
American Society for Aesthetic Plastic Surgery, 36, 51
American Society of Plastic Surgeons, 4–5, 7, 9, 12, 13, 15, 17, 19, 21, 22, 23, 24, 33, 34, 36, 38
American Urological Association, 50, 51
anaplastic large cell lymphoma, 11–12
anesthesia, reactions to, 42, 45–46, 53
augmentation, breast, 7, 9–12, 25, 31, 33, 38, 47–48, 52

B

before-and-after pictures, 34
body dysmorphic disorder, 27
Botox, 20–21, 24
breast jobs, 7, 9–12, 17, 19, 25, 31, 33, 38, 47–48, 52

C

California State Medical Board, 49
cancer, 10, 11, 48
capsular contracture, 47
carbolic acid, 22
cardiac arrest, 43, 50, 53
cardiac arrhythmia, 43
certification, doctors', 4, 34–36, 37, 38, 39
chemical peels, 9, 22
clinical trials, 11
collagen injections, 17, 23, 29, 51–52
congenital defects, 5
cosmetic surgery
  common procedures, 7, 9–23, 33
  major issues, 32–38
  myths and facts, 24
  outpatient, 44–46
  overview, 4–8
  parents' role, 29–31, 40
  questions to ask a doctor, 39–40
  risks and dangers, 16, 24, 25, 32, 34, 36, 38, 41–54
  why people get it, 5, 7, 15, 20, 25–31, 53

D

dermabrasion, 9, 15, 48–49
dermaplaning, 15
dermatone, 15
diet, 53

E

ear surgery, 7, 9, 16–17
eating disorders, 29
ectropion, 47

About the Authors

Nellie Vlad is a writer who lives in Alexandria, Virginia.

Frances O'Connor is a former New York City school teacher and the author of several books for young adults. She now lives in Albany, New York.

Photo Credits

Cover Floresco Productions/OJO Images/Getty Images; p. 6 Monica Rodriguez/Digital Vision/Getty Images; p. 10 Nucleus Medical Art, Inc./Collection Mix: Subjects/Getty Images; pp. 13 (top), 21 Shutterstock.com; p. 13 (bottom) Image Source/Getty Images; p. 18 Treible/Newscom; p. 26 Karan Kapoor/Stone/Getty Images; p. 28 Lucas Jackson/Reuters/Landov; p. 30 Alex Martin Photographers/Johner Images/Getty Images; p. 33 © Warner Bros. Television/Courtesy Everett Collection; p. 35 Adam Gault/Science Photo Library/Getty Images; p. 37 Wendy Hope/Stockbyte/Thinkstock; p. 42 Dominique Faget/AFP/Getty Images; p. 45 Thomas Barwick/The Image Bank/Getty Images; p. 46 © www.istockphoto.com/Jodi Jacobson; p. 51 Jason LaVeris/FilmMagic/Getty Images; p. 54 © Robin Nelson/PhotoEdit.

Designer: Les Kanturek; Photo Researcher: Karen Huang